SUCCESS is a STATE of MIND

This Journal Belongs To

Title ....

Name ....

What is the 75 Hard challenge Book?

The 75 hard challenge is a concept that was made to change your physical and mental health, therefore, change your life for the better through mental toughness.

The challenge consists of sticking to certain principles for 75 days non-stop. These basic pillars or principles are:

1. Follow a diet. The challenge doesn't specify or choose a specific diet for you. It is for you to plan! Although, the diet must exclude alcohol or cheat meals.

2. Workout twice a day for at least 45 minutes. The challenge dictates that it is better for one of these workouts to be an outdoor session.

3. Drink 4 liters of water.

4. Read 10 pages of a book every day.

5. Take five minutes cold shower.

6. Take a progress photo daily.

7. Perform one act of kindness.

How to use this journal?

It is very simple and easy to use. Before you start every day, write the day number in the circle (check 6).

Each day you will have to fill-in two pages (ex: pages 8 and 9).

The first page helps you organizing your day via daily schedule and to do list. You can also tracks your achievement by the end of the day using the daily check-list.

The second page contains details about your diet planning, and workout strategy, and all the other principles you have to stick to during the challenge.

That's just it... Have fun !!!

The 75 Hard Challenge

START DATE:

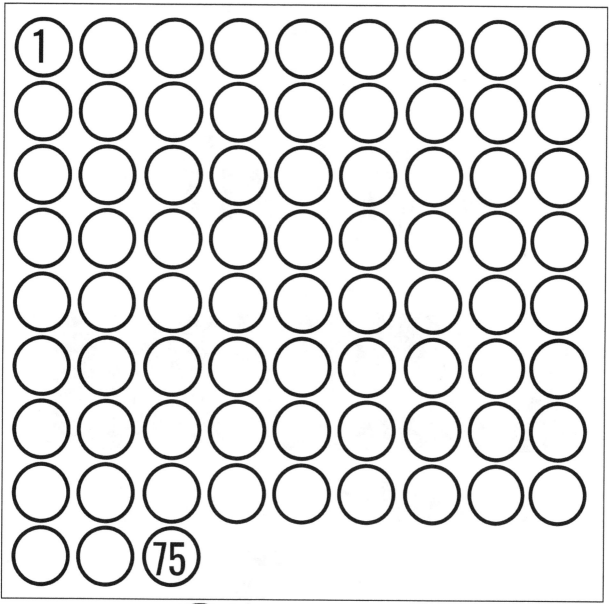

WEIGHT GOAL:

AFFIRMATION:

SUCCESS
is getting what you
★ WANT ★

Happiness

is wanting what you
GET

DATE: .... # Daily Schedule   DAY 1

DAILY SCHEDULE

6:00 am
7:00 am
8:00 am
9:00 am
10:00 am
11:00 am
12:00 am
13:00 pm
14:00 pm
15:00 pm
16:00 pm
17:00 pm
18:00 pm
19:00 pm
20:00 pm
21:00 pm
22:00 pm

DAILY CHECK LIST

- ○ FOLLOW A DIET
- ○ 45 Min WORKOUT
- ○ 4 LITRES WATER
- ○ 10 PAGES READING
- ○ 5 Min COLD SHOWER
- ○ NO ALCOHOL & CHEAT MEAL
- ○ ONE ACT OF KINDNESS

TO DO LIST

- ○
- ○
- ○
- ○
- ○
- ○
- ○
- ○
- ○
- ○
- ○
- ○

DIET PLAN

BREAKFAST	
LUNCH	
DINNER	

WORKOUT PLAN

EXERCISE	REPETITION	DURATION	NOTES

READING

TITLE	AUTHOR	PAGES

MOOD TRACKER

☺ ☺ ☹ 😠
☐ ☐ ☐ ☐

WATER INTAKE

1L ☐ 1L ☐ 1L ☐ 1L ☐

AN ACT OF KINDNESS I DID TODAY:

DATE: .... # Daily Schedule

DAILY SCHEDULE

- 6:00 am
- 7:00 am
- 8:00 am
- 9:00 am
- 10:00 am
- 11:00 am
- 12:00 am
- 13:00 pm
- 14:00 pm
- 15:00 pm
- 16:00 pm
- 17:00 pm
- 18:00 pm
- 19:00 pm
- 20:00 pm
- 21:00 pm
- 22:00 pm

DAILY CHECK LIST

- ○ FOLLOW A DIET
- ○ 45 Min WORKOUT
- ○ 4 LITRES WATER
- ○ 10 PAGES READING
- ○ 5 Min COLD SHOWER
- ○ NO ALCOHOL & CHEAT MEAL
- ○ ONE ACT OF KINDNESS

TO DO LIST

- ○
- ○
- ○
- ○
- ○
- ○
- ○
- ○
- ○
- ○
- ○
- ○

DIET PLAN		
	BREAKFAST	
	LUNCH	
	DINNER	

WORKOUT PLAN				
	EXERCISE	REPETITION	DURATION	NOTES

READING			
	TITLE	AUTHOR	PAGES

MOOD TRACKER

WATER INTAKE

AN ACT OF KINDNESS I DID TODAY:

DATE: _____ # Daily Schedule

DAILY SCHEDULE

- 6:00 am
- 7:00 am
- 8:00 am
- 9:00 am
- 10:00 am
- 11:00 am
- 12:00 am
- 13:00 pm
- 14:00 pm
- 15:00 pm
- 16:00 pm
- 17:00 pm
- 18:00 pm
- 19:00 pm
- 20:00 pm
- 21:00 pm
- 22:00 pm

DAILY CHECK LIST

- ○ FOLLOW A DIET
- ○ 45 Min WORKOUT
- ○ 4 LITRES WATER
- ○ 10 PAGES READING
- ○ 5 Min COLD SHOWER
- ○ NO ALCOHOL & CHEAT MEAL
- ○ ONE ACT OF KINDNESS

TO DO LIST

- ○
- ○
- ○
- ○
- ○
- ○
- ○
- ○
- ○
- ○
- ○

DIET PLAN

BREAKFAST	
LUNCH	
DINNER	

WORKOUT PLAN

EXERCISE	REPETITION	DURATION	NOTES

READING

TITLE	AUTHOR	PAGES

MOOD TRACKER

WATER INTAKE

AN ACT OF KINDNESS I DID TODAY:

DATE: .... # Daily Schedule

DAILY SCHEDULE

6:00 am
7:00 am
8:00 am
9:00 am
10:00 am
11:00 am
12:00 am
13:00 pm
14:00 pm
15:00 pm
16:00 pm
17:00 pm
18:00 pm
19:00 pm
20:00 pm
21:00 pm
22:00 pm

DAILY CHECK LIST

○ FOLLOW A DIET
○ 45 Min WORKOUT
○ 4 LITRES WATER
○ 10 PAGES READING
○ 5 Min COLD SHOWER
○ NO ALCOHOL & CHEAT MEAL
○ ONE ACT OF KINDNESS

TO DO LIST

○
○
○
○
○
○
○
○
○
○
○
○

DIET PLAN

BREAKFAST	
LUNCH	
DINNER	

WORKOUT PLAN

EXERCISE	REPETITION	DURATION	NOTES

READING

TITLE	AUTHOR	PAGES

MOOD TRACKER

WATER INTAKE

AN ACT OF KINDNESS I DID TODAY:

Daily Schedule

DATE: ....

DAILY SCHEDULE

- 6:00 am
- 7:00 am
- 8:00 am
- 9:00 am
- 10:00 am
- 11:00 am
- 12:00 am
- 13:00 pm
- 14:00 pm
- 15:00 pm
- 16:00 pm
- 17:00 pm
- 18:00 pm
- 19:00 pm
- 20:00 pm
- 21:00 pm
- 22:00 pm

DAILY CHECK LIST

- ○ FOLLOW A DIET
- ○ 45 Min WORKOUT
- ○ 4 LITRES WATER
- ○ 10 PAGES READING
- ○ 5 Min COLD SHOWER
- ○ NO ALCOHOL & CHEAT MEAL
- ○ ONE ACT OF KINDNESS

TO DO LIST

- ○
- ○
- ○
- ○
- ○
- ○
- ○
- ○
- ○
- ○
- ○
- ○

DIET PLAN		
	BREAKFAST	
	LUNCH	
	DINNER	

WORKOUT PLAN				
	EXERCISE	REPETITION	DURATION	NOTES

READING			
	TITLE	AUTHOR	PAGES

MOOD TRACKER

WATER INTAKE

AN ACT OF KINDNESS I DID TODAY:

DATE: .... # Daily Schedule

DAILY SCHEDULE

- 6:00 am
- 7:00 am
- 8:00 am
- 9:00 am
- 10:00 am
- 11:00 am
- 12:00 am
- 13:00 pm
- 14:00 pm
- 15:00 pm
- 16:00 pm
- 17:00 pm
- 18:00 pm
- 19:00 pm
- 20:00 pm
- 21:00 pm
- 22:00 pm

DAILY CHECK LIST

- ○ FOLLOW A DIET
- ○ 45 Min WORKOUT
- ○ 4 LITRES WATER
- ○ 10 PAGES READING
- ○ 5 Min COLD SHOWER
- ○ NO ALCOHOL & CHEAT MEAL
- ○ ONE ACT OF KINDNESS

TO DO LIST

- ○
- ○
- ○
- ○
- ○
- ○
- ○
- ○
- ○
- ○
- ○
- ○

DIET PLAN		
	BREAKFAST	
	LUNCH	
	DINNER	

WORKOUT PLAN				
	EXERCISE	REPETITION	DURATION	NOTES

READING			
	TITLE	AUTHOR	PAGES

MOOD TRACKER

WATER INTAKE

AN ACT OF KINDNESS I DID TODAY:

DATE: ....

Daily Schedule

 DAY 7

DAILY SCHEDULE

- 6:00 am
- 7:00 am
- 8:00 am
- 9:00 am
- 10:00 am
- 11:00 am
- 12:00 am
- 13:00 pm
- 14:00 pm
- 15:00 pm
- 16:00 pm
- 17:00 pm
- 18:00 pm
- 19:00 pm
- 20:00 pm
- 21:00 pm
- 22:00 pm

DAILY CHECK LIST

- ○ FOLLOW A DIET
- ○ 45 Min WORKOUT
- ○ 4 LITRES WATER
- ○ 10 PAGES READING
- ○ 5 Min COLD SHOWER
- ○ NO ALCOHOL & CHEAT MEAL
- ○ ONE ACT OF KINDNESS

TO DO LIST

- ○
- ○
- ○
- ○
- ○
- ○
- ○
- ○
- ○
- ○
- ○
- ○

DIET PLAN

BREAKFAST	
LUNCH	
DINNER	

WORKOUT PLAN

EXERCISE	REPETITION	DURATION	NOTES

READING

TITLE	AUTHOR	PAGES

MOOD TRACKER

WATER INTAKE

1L 1L 1L 1L

AN ACT OF KINDNESS I DID TODAY:

DATE: _____ # Daily Schedule

DAILY SCHEDULE

- 6:00 am
- 7:00 am
- 8:00 am
- 9:00 am
- 10:00 am
- 11:00 am
- 12:00 am
- 13:00 pm
- 14:00 pm
- 15:00 pm
- 16:00 pm
- 17:00 pm
- 18:00 pm
- 19:00 pm
- 20:00 pm
- 21:00 pm
- 22:00 pm

DAILY CHECK LIST

- ○ FOLLOW A DIET
- ○ 45 Min WORKOUT
- ○ 4 LITRES WATER
- ○ 10 PAGES READING
- ○ 5 Min COLD SHOWER
- ○ NO ALCOHOL & CHEAT MEAL
- ○ ONE ACT OF KINDNESS

TO DO LIST

- ○
- ○
- ○
- ○
- ○
- ○
- ○
- ○
- ○
- ○
- ○
- ○

DIET PLAN		
	BREAKFAST	
	LUNCH	
	DINNER	

WORKOUT PLAN			
EXERCISE	REPETITION	DURATION	NOTES

READING		
TITLE	AUTHOR	PAGES

MOOD TRACKER

WATER INTAKE

AN ACT OF KINDNESS I DID TODAY:

DATE: .... # Daily Schedule   DAY 9

DAILY SCHEDULE

- 6:00 am
- 7:00 am
- 8:00 am
- 9:00 am
- 10:00 am
- 11:00 am
- 12:00 am
- 13:00 pm
- 14:00 pm
- 15:00 pm
- 16:00 pm
- 17:00 pm
- 18:00 pm
- 19:00 pm
- 20:00 pm
- 21:00 pm
- 22:00 pm

DAILY CHECK LIST

- ○ FOLLOW A DIET
- ○ 45 Min WORKOUT
- ○ 4 LITRES WATER
- ○ 10 PAGES READING
- ○ 5 Min COLD SHOWER
- ○ NO ALCOHOL & CHEAT MEAL
- ○ ONE ACT OF KINDNESS

TO DO LIST

- ○
- ○
- ○
- ○
- ○
- ○
- ○
- ○
- ○
- ○
- ○

DIET PLAN

BREAKFAST	
LUNCH	
DINNER	

WORKOUT PLAN

EXERCISE	REPETITION	DURATION	NOTES

READING

TITLE	AUTHOR	PAGES

MOOD TRACKER

WATER INTAKE

AN ACT OF KINDNESS I DID TODAY:

Daily Schedule

DATE: ....

DAY 10

DAILY SCHEDULE

- 6:00 am
- 7:00 am
- 8:00 am
- 9:00 am
- 10:00 am
- 11:00 am
- 12:00 am
- 13:00 pm
- 14:00 pm
- 15:00 pm
- 16:00 pm
- 17:00 pm
- 18:00 pm
- 19:00 pm
- 20:00 pm
- 21:00 pm
- 22:00 pm

DAILY CHECK LIST

- ○ FOLLOW A DIET
- ○ 45 Min WORKOUT
- ○ 4 LITRES WATER
- ○ 10 PAGES READING
- ○ 5 Min COLD SHOWER
- ○ NO ALCOHOL & CHEAT MEAL
- ○ ONE ACT OF KINDNESS

TO DO LIST

- ○
- ○
- ○
- ○
- ○
- ○
- ○
- ○
- ○
- ○
- ○
- ○

DIET PLAN

BREAKFAST	
LUNCH	
DINNER	

WORKOUT PLAN

EXERCISE	REPETITION	DURATION	NOTES

READING

TITLE	AUTHOR	PAGES

MOOD TRACKER

WATER INTAKE

AN ACT OF KINDNESS I DID TODAY:

DATE: ....

Daily Schedule

DAY 11

DAILY SCHEDULE

6:00 am
7:00 am
8:00 am
9:00 am
10:00 am
11:00 am
12:00 am
13:00 pm
14:00 pm
15:00 pm
16:00 pm
17:00 pm
18:00 pm
19:00 pm
20:00 pm
21:00 pm
22:00 pm

DAILY CHECK LIST

- ○ FOLLOW A DIET
- ○ 45 Min WORKOUT
- ○ 4 LITRES WATER
- ○ 10 PAGES READING
- ○ 5 Min COLD SHOWER
- ○ NO ALCOHOL & CHEAT MEAL
- ○ ONE ACT OF KINDNESS

TO DO LIST

- ○
- ○
- ○
- ○
- ○
- ○
- ○
- ○
- ○
- ○
- ○
- ○

DIET PLAN

BREAKFAST	
LUNCH	
DINNER	

WORKOUT PLAN

EXERCISE	REPETITION	DURATION	NOTES

READING

TITLE	AUTHOR	PAGES

MOOD TRACKER

WATER INTAKE

AN ACT OF KINDNESS I DID TODAY:

DATE: _____ # Daily Schedule   **DAY 12**

DAILY SCHEDULE

6:00 am
7:00 am
8:00 am
9:00 am
10:00 am
11:00 am
12:00 am
13:00 pm
14:00 pm
15:00 pm
16:00 pm
17:00 pm
18:00 pm
19:00 pm
20:00 pm
21:00 pm
22:00 pm

DAILY CHECK LIST

- ○ FOLLOW A DIET
- ○ 45 Min WORKOUT
- ○ 4 LITRES WATER
- ○ 10 PAGES READING
- ○ 5 Min COLD SHOWER
- ○ NO ALCOHOL & CHEAT MEAL
- ○ ONE ACT OF KINDNESS

TO DO LIST

- ○
- ○
- ○
- ○
- ○
- ○
- ○
- ○
- ○
- ○
- ○
- ○

DIET PLAN

BREAKFAST	
LUNCH	
DINNER	

WORKOUT PLAN

EXERCISE	REPETITION	DURATION	NOTES

READING

TITLE	AUTHOR	PAGES

MOOD TRACKER

WATER INTAKE

AN ACT OF KINDNESS I DID TODAY:

DATE: ....

Daily Schedule

 DAY 13

DAILY SCHEDULE

6:00 am
7:00 am
8:00 am
9:00 am
10:00 am
11:00 am
12:00 am
13:00 pm
14:00 pm
15:00 pm
16:00 pm
17:00 pm
18:00 pm
19:00 pm
20:00 pm
21:00 pm
22:00 pm

DAILY CHECK LIST

○ FOLLOW A DIET
○ 45 Min WORKOUT
○ 4 LITRES WATER
○ 10 PAGES READING
○ 5 Min COLD SHOWER
○ NO ALCOHOL & CHEAT MEAL
○ ONE ACT OF KINDNESS

TO DO LIST

○
○
○
○
○
○
○
○
○
○
○
○

DIET PLAN		
	BREAKFAST	
	LUNCH	
	DINNER	

WORKOUT PLAN				
	EXERCISE	REPETITION	DURATION	NOTES

READING			
	TITLE	AUTHOR	PAGES

MOOD TRACKER

WATER INTAKE

AN ACT OF KINDNESS I DID TODAY:

DATE: ....

Daily Schedule

DAY 14

DAILY SCHEDULE

6:00 am
7:00 am
8:00 am
9:00 am
10:00 am
11:00 am
12:00 am
13:00 pm
14:00 pm
15:00 pm
16:00 pm
17:00 pm
18:00 pm
19:00 pm
20:00 pm
21:00 pm
22:00 pm

DAILY CHECK LIST

- ○ FOLLOW A DIET
- ○ 45 Min WORKOUT
- ○ 4 LITRES WATER
- ○ 10 PAGES READING
- ○ 5 Min COLD SHOWER
- ○ NO ALCOHOL & CHEAT MEAL
- ○ ONE ACT OF KINDNESS

TO DO LIST

○
○
○
○
○
○
○
○
○
○
○
○
○

DIET PLAN

BREAKFAST	
LUNCH	
DINNER	

WORKOUT PLAN

EXERCISE	REPETITION	DURATION	NOTES

READING

TITLE	AUTHOR	PAGES

MOOD TRACKER

WATER INTAKE

AN ACT OF KINDNESS I DID TODAY:

DATE: .... # Daily Schedule   DAY 15

DAILY SCHEDULE

- 6:00 am
- 7:00 am
- 8:00 am
- 9:00 am
- 10:00 am
- 11:00 am
- 12:00 am
- 13:00 pm
- 14:00 pm
- 15:00 pm
- 16:00 pm
- 17:00 pm
- 18:00 pm
- 19:00 pm
- 20:00 pm
- 21:00 pm
- 22:00 pm

DAILY CHECK LIST

- ○ FOLLOW A DIET
- ○ 45 Min WORKOUT
- ○ 4 LITRES WATER
- ○ 10 PAGES READING
- ○ 5 Min COLD SHOWER
- ○ NO ALCOHOL & CHEAT MEAL
- ○ ONE ACT OF KINDNESS

TO DO LIST

- ○
- ○
- ○
- ○
- ○
- ○
- ○
- ○
- ○
- ○
- ○
- ○

DIET PLAN

BREAKFAST	
LUNCH	
DINNER	

WORKOUT PLAN

EXERCISE	REPETITION	DURATION	NOTES

READING

TITLE	AUTHOR	PAGES

MOOD TRACKER

WATER INTAKE

AN ACT OF KINDNESS I DID TODAY:

DATE: _____   # Daily Schedule   **DAY 16**

DAILY SCHEDULE

- 6:00 am ....
- 7:00 am ....
- 8:00 am ....
- 9:00 am ....
- 10:00 am ....
- 11:00 am ....
- 12:00 am ....
- 13:00 pm ....
- 14:00 pm ....
- 15:00 pm ....
- 16:00 pm ....
- 17:00 pm ....
- 18:00 pm ....
- 19:00 pm ....
- 20:00 pm ....
- 21:00 pm ....
- 22:00 pm ....

DAILY CHECK LIST

- ○ FOLLOW A DIET
- ○ 45 Min WORKOUT
- ○ 4 LITRES WATER
- ○ 10 PAGES READING
- ○ 5 Min COLD SHOWER
- ○ NO ALCOHOL & CHEAT MEAL
- ○ ONE ACT OF KINDNESS

TO DO LIST

- ○ ....
- ○ ....
- ○ ....
- ○ ....
- ○ ....
- ○ ....
- ○ ....
- ○ ....
- ○ ....
- ○ ....
- ○ ....
- ○ ....

DIET PLAN

BREAKFAST		
LUNCH		
DINNER		

WORKOUT PLAN

EXERCISE	REPETITION	DURATION	NOTES

READING

TITLE	AUTHOR	PAGES

MOOD TRACKER

WATER INTAKE

AN ACT OF KINDNESS I DID TODAY:

DATE: ....

Daily Schedule

DAY 17

DAILY SCHEDULE

6:00 am ....
7:00 am ....
8:00 am ....
9:00 am ....
10:00 am ....
11:00 am ....
12:00 am ....
13:00 pm ....
14:00 pm ....
15:00 pm ....
16:00 pm ....
17:00 pm ....
18:00 pm ....
19:00 pm ....
20:00 pm ....
21:00 pm ....
22:00 pm ....

DAILY CHECK LIST

○ FOLLOW A DIET
○ 45 Min WORKOUT
○ 4 LITRES WATER
○ 10 PAGES READING
○ 5 Min COLD SHOWER
○ NO ALCOHOL & CHEAT MEAL
○ ONE ACT OF KINDNESS

TO DO LIST

○ ....
○ ....
○ ....
○ ....
○ ....
○ ....
○ ....
○ ....
○ ....
○ ....
○ ....
○ ....

DIET PLAN		
	BREAKFAST	
	LUNCH	
	DINNER	

WORKOUT PLAN				
	EXERCISE	REPETITION	DURATION	NOTES

READING			
	TITLE	AUTHOR	PAGES

MOOD TRACKER

WATER INTAKE

AN ACT OF KINDNESS I DID TODAY:

DATE: .... # Daily Schedule   DAY 18

DAILY SCHEDULE

6:00 am
7:00 am
8:00 am
9:00 am
10:00 am
11:00 am
12:00 am
13:00 pm
14:00 pm
15:00 pm
16:00 pm
17:00 pm
18:00 pm
19:00 pm
20:00 pm
21:00 pm
22:00 pm

DAILY CHECK LIST

- ◯ FOLLOW A DIET
- ◯ 45 Min WORKOUT
- ◯ 4 LITRES WATER
- ◯ 10 PAGES READING
- ◯ 5 Min COLD SHOWER
- ◯ NO ALCOHOL & CHEAT MEAL
- ◯ ONE ACT OF KINDNESS

TO DO LIST

- ◯
- ◯
- ◯
- ◯
- ◯
- ◯
- ◯
- ◯
- ◯
- ◯
- ◯
- ◯

DIET PLAN

BREAKFAST	
LUNCH	
DINNER	

WORKOUT PLAN

EXERCISE	REPETITION	DURATION	NOTES

READING

TITLE	AUTHOR	PAGES

MOOD TRACKER

WATER INTAKE

AN ACT OF KINDNESS I DID TODAY:

DATE: .... # Daily Schedule

DAILY SCHEDULE

- 6:00 am
- 7:00 am
- 8:00 am
- 9:00 am
- 10:00 am
- 11:00 am
- 12:00 am
- 13:00 pm
- 14:00 pm
- 15:00 pm
- 16:00 pm
- 17:00 pm
- 18:00 pm
- 19:00 pm
- 20:00 pm
- 21:00 pm
- 22:00 pm

DAILY CHECK LIST

- ○ FOLLOW A DIET
- ○ 45 Min WORKOUT
- ○ 4 LITRES WATER
- ○ 10 PAGES READING
- ○ 5 Min COLD SHOWER
- ○ NO ALCOHOL & CHEAT MEAL
- ○ ONE ACT OF KINDNESS

TO DO LIST

- ○
- ○
- ○
- ○
- ○
- ○
- ○
- ○
- ○
- ○
- ○
- ○

DIET PLAN		
	BREAKFAST	
	LUNCH	
	DINNER	

WORKOUT PLAN				
	EXERCISE	REPETITION	DURATION	NOTES

READING			
	TITLE	AUTHOR	PAGES

MOOD TRACKER

WATER INTAKE

AN ACT OF KINDNESS I DID TODAY:

DATE: _____ # Daily Schedule DAY 20

DAILY SCHEDULE

6:00 am
7:00 am
8:00 am
9:00 am
10:00 am
11:00 am
12:00 am
13:00 pm
14:00 pm
15:00 pm
16:00 pm
17:00 pm
18:00 pm
19:00 pm
20:00 pm
21:00 pm
22:00 pm

DAILY CHECK LIST

○ FOLLOW A DIET
○ 45 Min WORKOUT
○ 4 LITRES WATER
○ 10 PAGES READING
○ 5 Min COLD SHOWER
○ NO ALCOHOL & CHEAT MEAL
○ ONE ACT OF KINDNESS

TO DO LIST

○
○
○
○
○
○
○
○
○
○
○
○

DIET PLAN

BREAKFAST	
LUNCH	
DINNER	

WORKOUT PLAN

EXERCISE	REPETITION	DURATION	NOTES

READING

TITLE	AUTHOR	PAGES

MOOD TRACKER

WATER INTAKE

AN ACT OF KINDNESS I DID TODAY:

DATE: _____

Daily Schedule

DAY 21

DAILY SCHEDULE

- 6:00 am
- 7:00 am
- 8:00 am
- 9:00 am
- 10:00 am
- 11:00 am
- 12:00 am
- 13:00 pm
- 14:00 pm
- 15:00 pm
- 16:00 pm
- 17:00 pm
- 18:00 pm
- 19:00 pm
- 20:00 pm
- 21:00 pm
- 22:00 pm

DAILY CHECK LIST

- ○ FOLLOW A DIET
- ○ 45 Min WORKOUT
- ○ 4 LITRES WATER
- ○ 10 PAGES READING
- ○ 5 Min COLD SHOWER
- ○ NO ALCOHOL & CHEAT MEAL
- ○ ONE ACT OF KINDNESS

TO DO LIST

- ○
- ○
- ○
- ○
- ○
- ○
- ○
- ○
- ○
- ○
- ○
- ○
- ○

DIET PLAN

BREAKFAST	
LUNCH	
DINNER	

WORKOUT PLAN

EXERCISE	REPETITION	DURATION	NOTES

READING

TITLE	AUTHOR	PAGES

MOOD TRACKER

WATER INTAKE

AN ACT OF KINDNESS I DID TODAY:

DATE: .... # Daily Schedule DAY 22

DAILY SCHEDULE

6:00 am
7:00 am
8:00 am
9:00 am
10:00 am
11:00 am
12:00 am
13:00 pm
14:00 pm
15:00 pm
16:00 pm
17:00 pm
18:00 pm
19:00 pm
20:00 pm
21:00 pm
22:00 pm

DAILY CHECK LIST

- ○ FOLLOW A DIET
- ○ 45 Min WORKOUT
- ○ 4 LITRES WATER
- ○ 10 PAGES READING
- ○ 5 Min COLD SHOWER
- ○ NO ALCOHOL & CHEAT MEAL
- ○ ONE ACT OF KINDNESS

TO DO LIST

○
○
○
○
○
○
○
○
○
○
○
○

50

DIET PLAN		
	BREAKFAST	
	LUNCH	
	DINNER	

WORKOUT PLAN				
	EXERCISE	REPETITION	DURATION	NOTES

READING			
	TITLE	AUTHOR	PAGES

MOOD TRACKER

WATER INTAKE

AN ACT OF KINDNESS I DID TODAY:

DATE: ....

Daily Schedule

DAY 23

DAILY SCHEDULE

6:00 am
7:00 am
8:00 am
9:00 am
10:00 am
11:00 am
12:00 am
13:00 pm
14:00 pm
15:00 pm
16:00 pm
17:00 pm
18:00 pm
19:00 pm
20:00 pm
21:00 pm
22:00 pm

DAILY CHECK LIST

○ FOLLOW A DIET
○ 45 Min WORKOUT
○ 4 LITRES WATER
○ 10 PAGES READING
○ 5 Min COLD SHOWER
○ NO ALCOHOL & CHEAT MEAL
○ ONE ACT OF KINDNESS

TO DO LIST

○
○
○
○
○
○
○
○
○
○
○
○

DIET PLAN

BREAKFAST	
LUNCH	
DINNER	

WORKOUT PLAN

EXERCISE	REPETITION	DURATION	NOTES

READING

TITLE	AUTHOR	PAGES

MOOD TRACKER

WATER INTAKE

AN ACT OF KINDNESS I DID TODAY:

DATE: .... # Daily Schedule **DAY 24**

DAILY SCHEDULE

- 6:00 am
- 7:00 am
- 8:00 am
- 9:00 am
- 10:00 am
- 11:00 am
- 12:00 am
- 13:00 pm
- 14:00 pm
- 15:00 pm
- 16:00 pm
- 17:00 pm
- 18:00 pm
- 19:00 pm
- 20:00 pm
- 21:00 pm
- 22:00 pm

DAILY CHECK LIST

- ○ FOLLOW A DIET
- ○ 45 Min WORKOUT
- ○ 4 LITRES WATER
- ○ 10 PAGES READING
- ○ 5 Min COLD SHOWER
- ○ NO ALCOHOL & CHEAT MEAL
- ○ ONE ACT OF KINDNESS

TO DO LIST

DIET PLAN

BREAKFAST	
LUNCH	
DINNER	

WORKOUT PLAN

EXERCISE	REPETITION	DURATION	NOTES

READING

TITLE	AUTHOR	PAGES

MOOD TRACKER

WATER INTAKE

AN ACT OF KINDNESS I DID TODAY:

DATE: _____ # Daily Schedule

DAILY SCHEDULE

- 6:00 am
- 7:00 am
- 8:00 am
- 9:00 am
- 10:00 am
- 11:00 am
- 12:00 am
- 13:00 pm
- 14:00 pm
- 15:00 pm
- 16:00 pm
- 17:00 pm
- 18:00 pm
- 19:00 pm
- 20:00 pm
- 21:00 pm
- 22:00 pm

DAILY CHECK LIST

- ○ FOLLOW A DIET
- ○ 45 Min WORKOUT
- ○ 4 LITRES WATER
- ○ 10 PAGES READING
- ○ 5 Min COLD SHOWER
- ○ NO ALCOHOL & CHEAT MEAL
- ○ ONE ACT OF KINDNESS

TO DO LIST

- ○
- ○
- ○
- ○
- ○
- ○
- ○
- ○
- ○
- ○
- ○
- ○

DIET PLAN		
	BREAKFAST	
	LUNCH	
	DINNER	

WORKOUT PLAN				
	EXERCISE	REPETITION	DURATION	NOTES

READING			
	TITLE	AUTHOR	PAGES

MOOD TRACKER

WATER INTAKE

AN ACT OF KINDNESS I DID TODAY:

DATE: ....

Daily Schedule

DAY 26

DAILY SCHEDULE

6:00 am
7:00 am
8:00 am
9:00 am
10:00 am
11:00 am
12:00 am
13:00 pm
14:00 pm
15:00 pm
16:00 pm
17:00 pm
18:00 pm
19:00 pm
20:00 pm
21:00 pm
22:00 pm

DAILY CHECK LIST

○ FOLLOW A DIET
○ 45 Min WORKOUT
○ 4 LITRES WATER
○ 10 PAGES READING
○ 5 Min COLD SHOWER
○ NO ALCOHOL & CHEAT MEAL
○ ONE ACT OF KINDNESS

TO DO LIST

○
○
○
○
○
○
○
○
○
○
○
○

58

DIET PLAN		
	BREAKFAST	
	LUNCH	
	DINNER	

WORKOUT PLAN	EXERCISE	REPETITION	DURATION	NOTES

READING	TITLE	AUTHOR	PAGES

MOOD TRACKER

WATER INTAKE

AN ACT OF KINDNESS I DID TODAY:

DATE: _____

Daily Schedule

DAY 27

DAILY SCHEDULE

- 6:00 am
- 7:00 am
- 8:00 am
- 9:00 am
- 10:00 am
- 11:00 am
- 12:00 am
- 13:00 pm
- 14:00 pm
- 15:00 pm
- 16:00 pm
- 17:00 pm
- 18:00 pm
- 19:00 pm
- 20:00 pm
- 21:00 pm
- 22:00 pm

DAILY CHECK LIST

- ○ FOLLOW A DIET
- ○ 45 Min WORKOUT
- ○ 4 LITRES WATER
- ○ 10 PAGES READING
- ○ 5 Min COLD SHOWER
- ○ NO ALCOHOL & CHEAT MEAL
- ○ ONE ACT OF KINDNESS

TO DO LIST

- ○
- ○
- ○
- ○
- ○
- ○
- ○
- ○
- ○
- ○
- ○
- ○
- ○

DIET PLAN

BREAKFAST	
LUNCH	
DINNER	

WORKOUT PLAN

EXERCISE	REPETITION	DURATION	NOTES

READING

TITLE	AUTHOR	PAGES

MOOD TRACKER

WATER INTAKE

AN ACT OF KINDNESS I DID TODAY:

DATE: ....

Daily Schedule

 DAY 28

DAILY SCHEDULE

6:00 am
7:00 am
8:00 am
9:00 am
10:00 am
11:00 am
12:00 am
13:00 pm
14:00 pm
15:00 pm
16:00 pm
17:00 pm
18:00 pm
19:00 pm
20:00 pm
21:00 pm
22:00 pm

DAILY CHECK LIST

- ○ FOLLOW A DIET
- ○ 45 Min WORKOUT
- ○ 4 LITRES WATER
- ○ 10 PAGES READING
- ○ 5 Min COLD SHOWER
- ○ NO ALCOHOL & CHEAT MEAL
- ○ ONE ACT OF KINDNESS

TO DO LIST

○
○
○
○
○
○
○
○
○
○
○
○

DIET PLAN		
	BREAKFAST	
	LUNCH	
	DINNER	

WORKOUT PLAN				
	EXERCISE	REPETITION	DURATION	NOTES

READING			
	TITLE	AUTHOR	PAGES

MOOD TRACKER

WATER INTAKE

AN ACT OF KINDNESS I DID TODAY:

DATE: ....

Daily Schedule

DAY 29

DAILY SCHEDULE

- 6:00 am
- 7:00 am
- 8:00 am
- 9:00 am
- 10:00 am
- 11:00 am
- 12:00 am
- 13:00 pm
- 14:00 pm
- 15:00 pm
- 16:00 pm
- 17:00 pm
- 18:00 pm
- 19:00 pm
- 20:00 pm
- 21:00 pm
- 22:00 pm

DAILY CHECK LIST

- ○ FOLLOW A DIET
- ○ 45 Min WORKOUT
- ○ 4 LITRES WATER
- ○ 10 PAGES READING
- ○ 5 Min COLD SHOWER
- ○ NO ALCOHOL & CHEAT MEAL
- ○ ONE ACT OF KINDNESS

TO DO LIST

- ○
- ○
- ○
- ○
- ○
- ○
- ○
- ○
- ○
- ○
- ○
- ○
- ○

DIET PLAN		
	BREAKFAST	
	LUNCH	
	DINNER	

WORKOUT PLAN				
	EXERCISE	REPETITION	DURATION	NOTES

READING			
	TITLE	AUTHOR	PAGES

MOOD TRACKER

WATER INTAKE

AN ACT OF KINDNESS I DID TODAY:

DATE: .... # Daily Schedule **DAY 30**

DAILY SCHEDULE

- 6:00 am ....
- 7:00 am ....
- 8:00 am ....
- 9:00 am ....
- 10:00 am ....
- 11:00 am ....
- 12:00 am ....
- 13:00 pm ....
- 14:00 pm ....
- 15:00 pm ....
- 16:00 pm ....
- 17:00 pm ....
- 18:00 pm ....
- 19:00 pm ....
- 20:00 pm ....
- 21:00 pm ....
- 22:00 pm ....

DAILY CHECK LIST

- ○ FOLLOW A DIET
- ○ 45 Min WORKOUT
- ○ 4 LITRES WATER
- ○ 10 PAGES READING
- ○ 5 Min COLD SHOWER
- ○ NO ALCOHOL & CHEAT MEAL
- ○ ONE ACT OF KINDNESS

TO DO LIST

- ○ ....
- ○ ....
- ○ ....
- ○ ....
- ○ ....
- ○ ....
- ○ ....
- ○ ....
- ○ ....
- ○ ....
- ○ ....
- ○ ....

DIET PLAN

BREAKFAST	
LUNCH	
DINNER	

WORKOUT PLAN

EXERCISE	REPETITION	DURATION	NOTES

READING

TITLE	AUTHOR	PAGES

MOOD TRACKER

WATER INTAKE

AN ACT OF KINDNESS I DID TODAY:

DATE: .... # Daily Schedule   DAY 31

DAILY SCHEDULE

6:00 am
7:00 am
8:00 am
9:00 am
10:00 am
11:00 am
12:00 am
13:00 pm
14:00 pm
15:00 pm
16:00 pm
17:00 pm
18:00 pm
19:00 pm
20:00 pm
21:00 pm
22:00 pm

DAILY CHECK LIST

- ○ FOLLOW A DIET
- ○ 45 Min WORKOUT
- ○ 4 LITRES WATER
- ○ 10 PAGES READING
- ○ 5 Min COLD SHOWER
- ○ NO ALCOHOL & CHEAT MEAL
- ○ ONE ACT OF KINDNESS

TO DO LIST

- ○
- ○
- ○
- ○
- ○
- ○
- ○
- ○
- ○
- ○
- ○
- ○
- ○

DIET PLAN

BREAKFAST	
LUNCH	
DINNER	

WORKOUT PLAN

EXERCISE	REPETITION	DURATION	NOTES

READING

TITLE	AUTHOR	PAGES

MOOD TRACKER

WATER INTAKE

AN ACT OF KINDNESS I DID TODAY:

Daily Schedule

DATE: ....

 DAY 32

DAILY SCHEDULE

- 6:00 am
- 7:00 am
- 8:00 am
- 9:00 am
- 10:00 am
- 11:00 am
- 12:00 am
- 13:00 pm
- 14:00 pm
- 15:00 pm
- 16:00 pm
- 17:00 pm
- 18:00 pm
- 19:00 pm
- 20:00 pm
- 21:00 pm
- 22:00 pm

DAILY CHECK LIST

- ○ FOLLOW A DIET
- ○ 45 Min WORKOUT
- ○ 4 LITRES WATER
- ○ 10 PAGES READING
- ○ 5 Min COLD SHOWER
- ○ NO ALCOHOL & CHEAT MEAL
- ○ ONE ACT OF KINDNESS

TO DO LIST

- ○
- ○
- ○
- ○
- ○
- ○
- ○
- ○
- ○
- ○
- ○
- ○

DIET PLAN

BREAKFAST	
LUNCH	
DINNER	

WORKOUT PLAN

EXERCISE	REPETITION	DURATION	NOTES

READING

TITLE	AUTHOR	PAGES

MOOD TRACKER

WATER INTAKE

AN ACT OF KINDNESS I DID TODAY:

DATE: ....

Daily Schedule

DAY 32

DAILY SCHEDULE

6:00 am
7:00 am
8:00 am
9:00 am
10:00 am
11:00 am
12:00 am
13:00 pm
14:00 pm
15:00 pm
16:00 pm
17:00 pm
18:00 pm
19:00 pm
20:00 pm
21:00 pm
22:00 pm

DAILY CHECK LIST

- ○ FOLLOW A DIET
- ○ 45 Min WORKOUT
- ○ 4 LITRES WATER
- ○ 10 PAGES READING
- ○ 5 Min COLD SHOWER
- ○ NO ALCOHOL & CHEAT MEAL
- ○ ONE ACT OF KINDNESS

TO DO LIST

○
○
○
○
○
○
○
○
○
○
○
○

DIET PLAN

BREAKFAST	
LUNCH	
DINNER	

WORKOUT PLAN

EXERCISE	REPETITION	DURATION	NOTES

READING

TITLE	AUTHOR	PAGES

MOOD TRACKER

WATER INTAKE

AN ACT OF KINDNESS I DID TODAY:

DATE: .... # Daily Schedule

DAILY SCHEDULE

- 6:00 am
- 7:00 am
- 8:00 am
- 9:00 am
- 10:00 am
- 11:00 am
- 12:00 am
- 13:00 pm
- 14:00 pm
- 15:00 pm
- 16:00 pm
- 17:00 pm
- 18:00 pm
- 19:00 pm
- 20:00 pm
- 21:00 pm
- 22:00 pm

DAILY CHECK LIST

- ○ FOLLOW A DIET
- ○ 45 Min WORKOUT
- ○ 4 LITRES WATER
- ○ 10 PAGES READING
- ○ 5 Min COLD SHOWER
- ○ NO ALCOHOL & CHEAT MEAL
- ○ ONE ACT OF KINDNESS

TO DO LIST

- ○
- ○
- ○
- ○
- ○
- ○
- ○
- ○
- ○
- ○
- ○
- ○
- ○

DIET PLAN

BREAKFAST	
LUNCH	
DINNER	

WORKOUT PLAN

EXERCISE	REPETITION	DURATION	NOTES

READING

TITLE	AUTHOR	PAGES

MOOD TRACKER

WATER INTAKE

AN ACT OF KINDNESS I DID TODAY:

DATE: ....

Daily Schedule

DAY 34

DAILY SCHEDULE

6:00 am
7:00 am
8:00 am
9:00 am
10:00 am
11:00 am
12:00 am
13:00 pm
14:00 pm
15:00 pm
16:00 pm
17:00 pm
18:00 pm
19:00 pm
20:00 pm
21:00 pm
22:00 pm

DAILY CHECK LIST

- ○ FOLLOW A DIET
- ○ 45 Min WORKOUT
- ○ 4 LITRES WATER
- ○ 10 PAGES READING
- ○ 5 Min COLD SHOWER
- ○ NO ALCOHOL & CHEAT MEAL
- ○ ONE ACT OF KINDNESS

TO DO LIST

- ○
- ○
- ○
- ○
- ○
- ○
- ○
- ○
- ○
- ○
- ○

DIET PLAN

BREAKFAST	
LUNCH	
DINNER	

WORKOUT PLAN

EXERCISE	REPETITION	DURATION	NOTES

READING

TITLE	AUTHOR	PAGES

MOOD TRACKER

WATER INTAKE

AN ACT OF KINDNESS I DID TODAY:

DATE: .... # Daily Schedule

DAILY SCHEDULE

- 6:00 am
- 7:00 am
- 8:00 am
- 9:00 am
- 10:00 am
- 11:00 am
- 12:00 am
- 13:00 pm
- 14:00 pm
- 15:00 pm
- 16:00 pm
- 17:00 pm
- 18:00 pm
- 19:00 pm
- 20:00 pm
- 21:00 pm
- 22:00 pm

DAILY CHECK LIST

- ○ FOLLOW A DIET
- ○ 45 Min WORKOUT
- ○ 4 LITRES WATER
- ○ 10 PAGES READING
- ○ 5 Min COLD SHOWER
- ○ NO ALCOHOL & CHEAT MEAL
- ○ ONE ACT OF KINDNESS

TO DO LIST

- ○
- ○
- ○
- ○
- ○
- ○
- ○
- ○
- ○
- ○
- ○
- ○

DIET PLAN

BREAKFAST	
LUNCH	
DINNER	

WORKOUT PLAN

EXERCISE	REPETITION	DURATION	NOTES

READING

TITLE	AUTHOR	PAGES

MOOD TRACKER

WATER INTAKE

AN ACT OF KINDNESS I DID TODAY:

DATE: _____ # Daily Schedule DAY 36

DAILY SCHEDULE

- 6:00 am
- 7:00 am
- 8:00 am
- 9:00 am
- 10:00 am
- 11:00 am
- 12:00 am
- 13:00 pm
- 14:00 pm
- 15:00 pm
- 16:00 pm
- 17:00 pm
- 18:00 pm
- 19:00 pm
- 20:00 pm
- 21:00 pm
- 22:00 pm

DAILY CHECK LIST

- ○ FOLLOW A DIET
- ○ 45 Min WORKOUT
- ○ 4 LITRES WATER
- ○ 10 PAGES READING
- ○ 5 Min COLD SHOWER
- ○ NO ALCOHOL & CHEAT MEAL
- ○ ONE ACT OF KINDNESS

TO DO LIST

- ○
- ○
- ○
- ○
- ○
- ○
- ○
- ○
- ○
- ○
- ○
- ○

DIET PLAN

BREAKFAST	
LUNCH	
DINNER	

WORKOUT PLAN

EXERCISE	REPETITION	DURATION	NOTES

READING

TITLE	AUTHOR	PAGES

MOOD TRACKER

WATER INTAKE

AN ACT OF KINDNESS I DID TODAY:

DATE: .... # Daily Schedule   DAY 37

DAILY SCHEDULE

- 6:00 am
- 7:00 am
- 8:00 am
- 9:00 am
- 10:00 am
- 11:00 am
- 12:00 am
- 13:00 pm
- 14:00 pm
- 15:00 pm
- 16:00 pm
- 17:00 pm
- 18:00 pm
- 19:00 pm
- 20:00 pm
- 21:00 pm
- 22:00 pm

DAILY CHECK LIST

- ○ FOLLOW A DIET
- ○ 45 Min WORKOUT
- ○ 4 LITRES WATER
- ○ 10 PAGES READING
- ○ 5 Min COLD SHOWER
- ○ NO ALCOHOL & CHEAT MEAL
- ○ ONE ACT OF KINDNESS

TO DO LIST

- ○
- ○
- ○
- ○
- ○
- ○
- ○
- ○
- ○
- ○
- ○

DIET PLAN

BREAKFAST	
LUNCH	
DINNER	

WORKOUT PLAN

EXERCISE	REPETITION	DURATION	NOTES

READING

TITLE	AUTHOR	PAGES

MOOD TRACKER

WATER INTAKE

AN ACT OF KINDNESS I DID TODAY:

DATE: ....

Daily Schedule

DAY 38

DAILY SCHEDULE

- 6:00 am
- 7:00 am
- 8:00 am
- 9:00 am
- 10:00 am
- 11:00 am
- 12:00 am
- 13:00 pm
- 14:00 pm
- 15:00 pm
- 16:00 pm
- 17:00 pm
- 18:00 pm
- 19:00 pm
- 20:00 pm
- 21:00 pm
- 22:00 pm

DAILY CHECK LIST

- ○ FOLLOW A DIET
- ○ 45 Min WORKOUT
- ○ 4 LITRES WATER
- ○ 10 PAGES READING
- ○ 5 Min COLD SHOWER
- ○ NO ALCOHOL & CHEAT MEAL
- ○ ONE ACT OF KINDNESS

TO DO LIST

- ○
- ○
- ○
- ○
- ○
- ○
- ○
- ○
- ○
- ○
- ○

DIET PLAN	BREAKFAST	
	LUNCH	
	DINNER	

	EXERCISE	REPETITION	DURATION	NOTES
WORKOUT PLAN				

	TITLE	AUTHOR	PAGES
READING			

MOOD TRACKER

WATER INTAKE

AN ACT OF KINDNESS I DID TODAY:

Daily Schedule

DATE: ....   **DAY 39**

DAILY SCHEDULE

- 6:00 am ....
- 7:00 am ....
- 8:00 am ....
- 9:00 am ....
- 10:00 am ....
- 11:00 am ....
- 12:00 am ....
- 13:00 pm ....
- 14:00 pm ....
- 15:00 pm ....
- 16:00 pm ....
- 17:00 pm ....
- 18:00 pm ....
- 19:00 pm ....
- 20:00 pm ....
- 21:00 pm ....
- 22:00 pm ....

DAILY CHECK LIST

- ○ FOLLOW A DIET
- ○ 45 Min WORKOUT
- ○ 4 LITRES WATER
- ○ 10 PAGES READING
- ○ 5 Min COLD SHOWER
- ○ NO ALCOHOL & CHEAT MEAL
- ○ ONE ACT OF KINDNESS

TO DO LIST

- ○ ....
- ○ ....
- ○ ....
- ○ ....
- ○ ....
- ○ ....
- ○ ....
- ○ ....
- ○ ....
- ○ ....

DIET PLAN

BREAKFAST	
LUNCH	
DINNER	

WORKOUT PLAN

EXERCISE	REPETITION	DURATION	NOTES

READING

TITLE	AUTHOR	PAGES

MOOD TRACKER

WATER INTAKE

1L 1L 1L 1L

AN ACT OF KINDNESS I DID TODAY:

DATE: ....

Daily Schedule

DAY 40

DAILY SCHEDULE

6:00 am
7:00 am
8:00 am
9:00 am
10:00 am
11:00 am
12:00 am
13:00 pm
14:00 pm
15:00 pm
16:00 pm
17:00 pm
18:00 pm
19:00 pm
20:00 pm
21:00 pm
22:00 pm

DAILY CHECK LIST

- ○ FOLLOW A DIET
- ○ 45 Min WORKOUT
- ○ 4 LITRES WATER
- ○ 10 PAGES READING
- ○ 5 Min COLD SHOWER
- ○ NO ALCOHOL & CHEAT MEAL
- ○ ONE ACT OF KINDNESS

TO DO LIST

- ○
- ○
- ○
- ○
- ○
- ○
- ○
- ○
- ○
- ○
- ○
- ○

DIET PLAN

BREAKFAST	
LUNCH	
DINNER	

WORKOUT PLAN

EXERCISE	REPETITION	DURATION	NOTES

READING

TITLE	AUTHOR	PAGES

MOOD TRACKER

WATER INTAKE

AN ACT OF KINDNESS I DID TODAY:

DATE: .... # Daily Schedule

DAILY SCHEDULE

- 6:00 am
- 7:00 am
- 8:00 am
- 9:00 am
- 10:00 am
- 11:00 am
- 12:00 am
- 13:00 pm
- 14:00 pm
- 15:00 pm
- 16:00 pm
- 17:00 pm
- 18:00 pm
- 19:00 pm
- 20:00 pm
- 21:00 pm
- 22:00 pm

DAILY CHECK LIST

- ○ FOLLOW A DIET
- ○ 45 Min WORKOUT
- ○ 4 LITRES WATER
- ○ 10 PAGES READING
- ○ 5 Min COLD SHOWER
- ○ NO ALCOHOL & CHEAT MEAL
- ○ ONE ACT OF KINDNESS

TO DO LIST

- ○
- ○
- ○
- ○
- ○
- ○
- ○
- ○
- ○
- ○
- ○

DIET PLAN		
	BREAKFAST	
	LUNCH	
	DINNER	

WORKOUT PLAN				
	EXERCISE	REPETITION	DURATION	NOTES

READING			
	TITLE	AUTHOR	PAGES

MOOD TRACKER

WATER INTAKE

AN ACT OF KINDNESS I DID TODAY:

DATE: _____

Daily Schedule

DAY 42

DAILY SCHEDULE

- 6:00 am
- 7:00 am
- 8:00 am
- 9:00 am
- 10:00 am
- 11:00 am
- 12:00 am
- 13:00 pm
- 14:00 pm
- 15:00 pm
- 16:00 pm
- 17:00 pm
- 18:00 pm
- 19:00 pm
- 20:00 pm
- 21:00 pm
- 22:00 pm

DAILY CHECK LIST

- ○ FOLLOW A DIET
- ○ 45 Min WORKOUT
- ○ 4 LITRES WATER
- ○ 10 PAGES READING
- ○ 5 Min COLD SHOWER
- ○ NO ALCOHOL & CHEAT MEAL
- ○ ONE ACT OF KINDNESS

TO DO LIST

- ○
- ○
- ○
- ○
- ○
- ○
- ○
- ○
- ○
- ○
- ○

DIET PLAN

BREAKFAST	
LUNCH	
DINNER	

WORKOUT PLAN

EXERCISE	REPETITION	DURATION	NOTES

READING

TITLE	AUTHOR	PAGES

MOOD TRACKER

WATER INTAKE

AN ACT OF KINDNESS I DID TODAY:

DATE: .... # Daily Schedule **DAY 43**

DAILY SCHEDULE

- 6:00 am
- 7:00 am
- 8:00 am
- 9:00 am
- 10:00 am
- 11:00 am
- 12:00 am
- 13:00 pm
- 14:00 pm
- 15:00 pm
- 16:00 pm
- 17:00 pm
- 18:00 pm
- 19:00 pm
- 20:00 pm
- 21:00 pm
- 22:00 pm

DAILY CHECK LIST

- ○ FOLLOW A DIET
- ○ 45 Min WORKOUT
- ○ 4 LITRES WATER
- ○ 10 PAGES READING
- ○ 5 Min COLD SHOWER
- ○ NO ALCOHOL & CHEAT MEAL
- ○ ONE ACT OF KINDNESS

TO DO LIST

- ○
- ○
- ○
- ○
- ○
- ○
- ○
- ○
- ○
- ○
- ○
- ○

DIET PLAN

BREAKFAST	
LUNCH	
DINNER	

WORKOUT PLAN

EXERCISE	REPETITION	DURATION	NOTES

READING

TITLE	AUTHOR	PAGES

MOOD TRACKER

WATER INTAKE

AN ACT OF KINDNESS I DID TODAY:

DATE: ....

Daily Schedule

DAY 44

DAILY SCHEDULE

- 6:00 am
- 7:00 am
- 8:00 am
- 9:00 am
- 10:00 am
- 11:00 am
- 12:00 am
- 13:00 pm
- 14:00 pm
- 15:00 pm
- 16:00 pm
- 17:00 pm
- 18:00 pm
- 19:00 pm
- 20:00 pm
- 21:00 pm
- 22:00 pm

DAILY CHECK LIST

- ○ FOLLOW A DIET
- ○ 45 Min WORKOUT
- ○ 4 LITRES WATER
- ○ 10 PAGES READING
- ○ 5 Min COLD SHOWER
- ○ NO ALCOHOL & CHEAT MEAL
- ○ ONE ACT OF KINDNESS

TO DO LIST

- ○
- ○
- ○
- ○
- ○
- ○
- ○
- ○
- ○
- ○
- ○
- ○

DIET PLAN		
	BREAKFAST	
	LUNCH	
	DINNER	

WORKOUT PLAN				
	EXERCISE	REPETITION	DURATION	NOTES

READING			
	TITLE	AUTHOR	PAGES

MOOD TRACKER

WATER INTAKE

AN ACT OF KINDNESS I DID TODAY:

DATE: .... # Daily Schedule   DAY 45

DAILY SCHEDULE

- 6:00 am
- 7:00 am
- 8:00 am
- 9:00 am
- 10:00 am
- 11:00 am
- 12:00 am
- 13:00 pm
- 14:00 pm
- 15:00 pm
- 16:00 pm
- 17:00 pm
- 18:00 pm
- 19:00 pm
- 20:00 pm
- 21:00 pm
- 22:00 pm

DAILY CHECK LIST

- ○ FOLLOW A DIET
- ○ 45 Min WORKOUT
- ○ 4 LITRES WATER
- ○ 10 PAGES READING
- ○ 5 Min COLD SHOWER
- ○ NO ALCOHOL & CHEAT MEAL
- ○ ONE ACT OF KINDNESS

TO DO LIST

- ○
- ○
- ○
- ○
- ○
- ○
- ○
- ○
- ○
- ○
- ○
- ○

DIET PLAN

BREAKFAST	
LUNCH	
DINNER	

WORKOUT PLAN

EXERCISE	REPETITION	DURATION	NOTES

READING

TITLE	AUTHOR	PAGES

MOOD TRACKER

WATER INTAKE

AN ACT OF KINDNESS I DID TODAY:

Daily Schedule

DATE: _____

 DAY 46

DAILY SCHEDULE

- 6:00 am
- 7:00 am
- 8:00 am
- 9:00 am
- 10:00 am
- 11:00 am
- 12:00 am
- 13:00 pm
- 14:00 pm
- 15:00 pm
- 16:00 pm
- 17:00 pm
- 18:00 pm
- 19:00 pm
- 20:00 pm
- 21:00 pm
- 22:00 pm

DAILY CHECK LIST

- ○ FOLLOW A DIET
- ○ 45 Min WORKOUT
- ○ 4 LITRES WATER
- ○ 10 PAGES READING
- ○ 5 Min COLD SHOWER
- ○ NO ALCOHOL & CHEAT MEAL
- ○ ONE ACT OF KINDNESS

TO DO LIST

- ○
- ○
- ○
- ○
- ○
- ○
- ○
- ○
- ○
- ○
- ○

DIET PLAN

BREAKFAST	
LUNCH	
DINNER	

WORKOUT PLAN

EXERCISE	REPETITION	DURATION	NOTES

READING

TITLE	AUTHOR	PAGES

MOOD TRACKER

WATER INTAKE

AN ACT OF KINDNESS I DID TODAY:

DATE: ....

Daily Schedule

DAY 47

DAILY SCHEDULE

- 6:00 am
- 7:00 am
- 8:00 am
- 9:00 am
- 10:00 am
- 11:00 am
- 12:00 am
- 13:00 pm
- 14:00 pm
- 15:00 pm
- 16:00 pm
- 17:00 pm
- 18:00 pm
- 19:00 pm
- 20:00 pm
- 21:00 pm
- 22:00 pm

DAILY CHECK LIST

- ○ FOLLOW A DIET
- ○ 45 Min WORKOUT
- ○ 4 LITRES WATER
- ○ 10 PAGES READING
- ○ 5 Min COLD SHOWER
- ○ NO ALCOHOL & CHEAT MEAL
- ○ ONE ACT OF KINDNESS

TO DO LIST

- ○
- ○
- ○
- ○
- ○
- ○
- ○
- ○
- ○
- ○
- ○

DIET PLAN	BREAKFAST	
	LUNCH	
	DINNER	

WORKOUT PLAN	EXERCISE	REPETITION	DURATION	NOTES

READING	TITLE	AUTHOR	PAGES

MOOD TRACKER

WATER INTAKE

AN ACT OF KINDNESS I DID TODAY:

DATE: _____

Daily Schedule

DAILY SCHEDULE

- 6:00 am
- 7:00 am
- 8:00 am
- 9:00 am
- 10:00 am
- 11:00 am
- 12:00 am
- 13:00 pm
- 14:00 pm
- 15:00 pm
- 16:00 pm
- 17:00 pm
- 18:00 pm
- 19:00 pm
- 20:00 pm
- 21:00 pm
- 22:00 pm

DAILY CHECK LIST

- ○ FOLLOW A DIET
- ○ 45 Min WORKOUT
- ○ 4 LITRES WATER
- ○ 10 PAGES READING
- ○ 5 Min COLD SHOWER
- ○ NO ALCOHOL & CHEAT MEAL
- ○ ONE ACT OF KINDNESS

TO DO LIST

- ○
- ○
- ○
- ○
- ○
- ○
- ○
- ○
- ○
- ○
- ○
- ○

DIET PLAN

BREAKFAST	
LUNCH	
DINNER	

WORKOUT PLAN

EXERCISE	REPETITION	DURATION	NOTES

READING

TITLE	AUTHOR	PAGES

MOOD TRACKER

WATER INTAKE

AN ACT OF KINDNESS I DID TODAY:

DATE: ....

Daily Schedule

DAILY SCHEDULE

- 6:00 am
- 7:00 am
- 8:00 am
- 9:00 am
- 10:00 am
- 11:00 am
- 12:00 am
- 13:00 pm
- 14:00 pm
- 15:00 pm
- 16:00 pm
- 17:00 pm
- 18:00 pm
- 19:00 pm
- 20:00 pm
- 21:00 pm
- 22:00 pm

DAILY CHECK LIST

- ○ FOLLOW A DIET
- ○ 45 Min WORKOUT
- ○ 4 LITRES WATER
- ○ 10 PAGES READING
- ○ 5 Min COLD SHOWER
- ○ NO ALCOHOL & CHEAT MEAL
- ○ ONE ACT OF KINDNESS

TO DO LIST

- ○
- ○
- ○
- ○
- ○
- ○
- ○
- ○
- ○
- ○
- ○
- ○

DIET PLAN		
	BREAKFAST	
	LUNCH	
	DINNER	

WORKOUT PLAN			
EXERCISE	REPETITION	DURATION	NOTES

READING		
TITLE	AUTHOR	PAGES

MOOD TRACKER

WATER INTAKE

AN ACT OF KINDNESS I DID TODAY:

DATE: ....

Daily Schedule

DAY 50

DAILY SCHEDULE

6:00 am
7:00 am
8:00 am
9:00 am
10:00 am
11:00 am
12:00 am
13:00 pm
14:00 pm
15:00 pm
16:00 pm
17:00 pm
18:00 pm
19:00 pm
20:00 pm
21:00 pm
22:00 pm

DAILY CHECK LIST

○ FOLLOW A DIET
○ 45 Min WORKOUT
○ 4 LITRES WATER
○ 10 PAGES READING
○ 5 Min COLD SHOWER
○ NO ALCOHOL & CHEAT MEAL
○ ONE ACT OF KINDNESS

TO DO LIST

○
○
○
○
○
○
○
○
○
○
○

DIET PLAN

BREAKFAST	
LUNCH	
DINNER	

WORKOUT PLAN

EXERCISE	REPETITION	DURATION	NOTES

READING

TITLE	AUTHOR	PAGES

MOOD TRACKER

WATER INTAKE

AN ACT OF KINDNESS I DID TODAY:

Daily Schedule

DATE: ....

 DAY 51

DAILY SCHEDULE

- 6:00 am
- 7:00 am
- 8:00 am
- 9:00 am
- 10:00 am
- 11:00 am
- 12:00 am
- 13:00 pm
- 14:00 pm
- 15:00 pm
- 16:00 pm
- 17:00 pm
- 18:00 pm
- 19:00 pm
- 20:00 pm
- 21:00 pm
- 22:00 pm

DAILY CHECK LIST

- ○ FOLLOW A DIET
- ○ 45 Min WORKOUT
- ○ 4 LITRES WATER
- ○ 10 PAGES READING
- ○ 5 Min COLD SHOWER
- ○ NO ALCOHOL & CHEAT MEAL
- ○ ONE ACT OF KINDNESS

TO DO LIST

- ○
- ○
- ○
- ○
- ○
- ○
- ○
- ○
- ○
- ○
- ○
- ○

DIET PLAN

BREAKFAST	
LUNCH	
DINNER	

WORKOUT PLAN

EXERCISE	REPETITION	DURATION	NOTES

READING

TITLE	AUTHOR	PAGES

MOOD TRACKER

WATER INTAKE

AN ACT OF KINDNESS I DID TODAY:

DATE: ....

Daily Schedule

DAY 52

DAILY SCHEDULE

- 6:00 am
- 7:00 am
- 8:00 am
- 9:00 am
- 10:00 am
- 11:00 am
- 12:00 am
- 13:00 pm
- 14:00 pm
- 15:00 pm
- 16:00 pm
- 17:00 pm
- 18:00 pm
- 19:00 pm
- 20:00 pm
- 21:00 pm
- 22:00 pm

DAILY CHECK LIST

- ○ FOLLOW A DIET
- ○ 45 Min WORKOUT
- ○ 4 LITRES WATER
- ○ 10 PAGES READING
- ○ 5 Min COLD SHOWER
- ○ NO ALCOHOL & CHEAT MEAL
- ○ ONE ACT OF KINDNESS

TO DO LIST

- ○
- ○
- ○
- ○
- ○
- ○
- ○
- ○
- ○
- ○
- ○
- ○

DIET PLAN

BREAKFAST	
LUNCH	
DINNER	

WORKOUT PLAN

EXERCISE	REPETITION	DURATION	NOTES

READING

TITLE	AUTHOR	PAGES

MOOD TRACKER

WATER INTAKE

AN ACT OF KINDNESS I DID TODAY:

DATE: ....

Daily Schedule

DAILY SCHEDULE

6:00 am
7:00 am
8:00 am
9:00 am
10:00 am
11:00 am
12:00 am
13:00 pm
14:00 pm
15:00 pm
16:00 pm
17:00 pm
18:00 pm
19:00 pm
20:00 pm
21:00 pm
22:00 pm

DAILY CHECK LIST

- ○ FOLLOW A DIET
- ○ 45 Min WORKOUT
- ○ 4 LITRES WATER
- ○ 10 PAGES READING
- ○ 5 Min COLD SHOWER
- ○ NO ALCOHOL & CHEAT MEAL
- ○ ONE ACT OF KINDNESS

TO DO LIST

- ○
- ○
- ○
- ○
- ○
- ○
- ○
- ○
- ○
- ○
- ○
- ○

DIET PLAN		
	BREAKFAST	
	LUNCH	
	DINNER	

WORKOUT PLAN			
EXERCISE	REPETITION	DURATION	NOTES

READING		
TITLE	AUTHOR	PAGES

MOOD TRACKER

WATER INTAKE

AN ACT OF KINDNESS I DID TODAY:

DATE: _____ # Daily Schedule

DAILY SCHEDULE

- 6:00 am
- 7:00 am
- 8:00 am
- 9:00 am
- 10:00 am
- 11:00 am
- 12:00 am
- 13:00 pm
- 14:00 pm
- 15:00 pm
- 16:00 pm
- 17:00 pm
- 18:00 pm
- 19:00 pm
- 20:00 pm
- 21:00 pm
- 22:00 pm

DAILY CHECK LIST

- ○ FOLLOW A DIET
- ○ 45 Min WORKOUT
- ○ 4 LITRES WATER
- ○ 10 PAGES READING
- ○ 5 Min COLD SHOWER
- ○ NO ALCOHOL & CHEAT MEAL
- ○ ONE ACT OF KINDNESS

TO DO LIST

DIET PLAN

BREAKFAST	
LUNCH	
DINNER	

WORKOUT PLAN

EXERCISE	REPETITION	DURATION	NOTES

READING

TITLE	AUTHOR	PAGES

MOOD TRACKER

WATER INTAKE

AN ACT OF KINDNESS I DID TODAY:

DATE: .... # Daily Schedule

DAILY SCHEDULE

- 6:00 am
- 7:00 am
- 8:00 am
- 9:00 am
- 10:00 am
- 11:00 am
- 12:00 am
- 13:00 pm
- 14:00 pm
- 15:00 pm
- 16:00 pm
- 17:00 pm
- 18:00 pm
- 19:00 pm
- 20:00 pm
- 21:00 pm
- 22:00 pm

DAILY CHECK LIST

- ○ FOLLOW A DIET
- ○ 45 Min WORKOUT
- ○ 4 LITRES WATER
- ○ 10 PAGES READING
- ○ 5 Min COLD SHOWER
- ○ NO ALCOHOL & CHEAT MEAL
- ○ ONE ACT OF KINDNESS

TO DO LIST

- ○
- ○
- ○
- ○
- ○
- ○
- ○
- ○
- ○
- ○
- ○
- ○

DIET PLAN

BREAKFAST	
LUNCH	
DINNER	

WORKOUT PLAN

EXERCISE	REPETITION	DURATION	NOTES

READING

TITLE	AUTHOR	PAGES

MOOD TRACKER

WATER INTAKE

AN ACT OF KINDNESS I DID TODAY:

DATE: .... # Daily Schedule   DAY 56

DAILY SCHEDULE

6:00 am
7:00 am
8:00 am
9:00 am
10:00 am
11:00 am
12:00 am
13:00 pm
14:00 pm
15:00 pm
16:00 pm
17:00 pm
18:00 pm
19:00 pm
20:00 pm
21:00 pm
22:00 pm

DAILY CHECK LIST

- ○ FOLLOW A DIET
- ○ 45 Min WORKOUT
- ○ 4 LITRES WATER
- ○ 10 PAGES READING
- ○ 5 Min COLD SHOWER
- ○ NO ALCOHOL & CHEAT MEAL
- ○ ONE ACT OF KINDNESS

TO DO LIST

- ○
- ○
- ○
- ○
- ○
- ○
- ○
- ○
- ○
- ○
- ○

DIET PLAN		
	BREAKFAST	
	LUNCH	
	DINNER	

WORKOUT PLAN				
	EXERCISE	REPETITION	DURATION	NOTES

READING			
	TITLE	AUTHOR	PAGES

MOOD TRACKER

WATER INTAKE

AN ACT OF KINDNESS I DID TODAY:

Daily Schedule

DATE: ....

DAY 57

DAILY SCHEDULE

- 6:00 am
- 7:00 am
- 8:00 am
- 9:00 am
- 10:00 am
- 11:00 am
- 12:00 am
- 13:00 pm
- 14:00 pm
- 15:00 pm
- 16:00 pm
- 17:00 pm
- 18:00 pm
- 19:00 pm
- 20:00 pm
- 21:00 pm
- 22:00 pm

DAILY CHECK LIST

- ○ FOLLOW A DIET
- ○ 45 Min WORKOUT
- ○ 4 LITRES WATER
- ○ 10 PAGES READING
- ○ 5 Min COLD SHOWER
- ○ NO ALCOHOL & CHEAT MEAL
- ○ ONE ACT OF KINDNESS

TO DO LIST

- ○
- ○
- ○
- ○
- ○
- ○
- ○
- ○
- ○
- ○
- ○

DIET PLAN

BREAKFAST	
LUNCH	
DINNER	

WORKOUT PLAN

EXERCISE	REPETITION	DURATION	NOTES

READING

TITLE	AUTHOR	PAGES

MOOD TRACKER

WATER INTAKE

AN ACT OF KINDNESS I DID TODAY:

DATE: _____

Daily Schedule

 DAY 58

DAILY SCHEDULE

- 6:00 am
- 7:00 am
- 8:00 am
- 9:00 am
- 10:00 am
- 11:00 am
- 12:00 am
- 13:00 pm
- 14:00 pm
- 15:00 pm
- 16:00 pm
- 17:00 pm
- 18:00 pm
- 19:00 pm
- 20:00 pm
- 21:00 pm
- 22:00 pm

DAILY CHECK LIST

- ○ FOLLOW A DIET
- ○ 45 Min WORKOUT
- ○ 4 LITRES WATER
- ○ 10 PAGES READING
- ○ 5 Min COLD SHOWER
- ○ NO ALCOHOL & CHEAT MEAL
- ○ ONE ACT OF KINDNESS

TO DO LIST

- ○
- ○
- ○
- ○
- ○
- ○
- ○
- ○
- ○
- ○
- ○
- ○

DIET PLAN

BREAKFAST	
LUNCH	
DINNER	

WORKOUT PLAN

EXERCISE	REPETITION	DURATION	NOTES

READING

TITLE	AUTHOR	PAGES

MOOD TRACKER

WATER INTAKE

1L 1L 1L 1L

AN ACT OF KINDNESS I DID TODAY:

DATE: ....   # Daily Schedule   DAY 59

DAILY SCHEDULE

- 6:00 am
- 7:00 am
- 8:00 am
- 9:00 am
- 10:00 am
- 11:00 am
- 12:00 am
- 13:00 pm
- 14:00 pm
- 15:00 pm
- 16:00 pm
- 17:00 pm
- 18:00 pm
- 19:00 pm
- 20:00 pm
- 21:00 pm
- 22:00 pm

DAILY CHECK LIST

- ○ FOLLOW A DIET
- ○ 45 Min WORKOUT
- ○ 4 LITRES WATER
- ○ 10 PAGES READING
- ○ 5 Min COLD SHOWER
- ○ NO ALCOHOL & CHEAT MEAL
- ○ ONE ACT OF KINDNESS

TO DO LIST

- ○
- ○
- ○
- ○
- ○
- ○
- ○
- ○
- ○
- ○
- ○
- ○

DIET PLAN

BREAKFAST	
LUNCH	
DINNER	

WORKOUT PLAN

EXERCISE	REPETITION	DURATION	NOTES

READING

TITLE	AUTHOR	PAGES

MOOD TRACKER

WATER INTAKE

1L 1L 1L 1L

AN ACT OF KINDNESS I DID TODAY:

DATE: ....

Daily Schedule

 DAY 60

DAILY SCHEDULE

- 6:00 am
- 7:00 am
- 8:00 am
- 9:00 am
- 10:00 am
- 11:00 am
- 12:00 am
- 13:00 pm
- 14:00 pm
- 15:00 pm
- 16:00 pm
- 17:00 pm
- 18:00 pm
- 19:00 pm
- 20:00 pm
- 21:00 pm
- 22:00 pm

DAILY CHECK LIST

- ○ FOLLOW A DIET
- ○ 45 Min WORKOUT
- ○ 4 LITRES WATER
- ○ 10 PAGES READING
- ○ 5 Min COLD SHOWER
- ○ NO ALCOHOL & CHEAT MEAL
- ○ ONE ACT OF KINDNESS

TO DO LIST

- ○
- ○
- ○
- ○
- ○
- ○
- ○
- ○
- ○
- ○
- ○
- ○

DIET PLAN	BREAKFAST	
	LUNCH	
	DINNER	

WORKOUT PLAN	EXERCISE	REPETITION	DURATION	NOTES

READING	TITLE	AUTHOR	PAGES

MOOD TRACKER

WATER INTAKE

AN ACT OF KINDNESS I DID TODAY:

DATE: .... # Daily Schedule   DAY 61

DAILY SCHEDULE

- 6:00 am
- 7:00 am
- 8:00 am
- 9:00 am
- 10:00 am
- 11:00 am
- 12:00 am
- 13:00 pm
- 14:00 pm
- 15:00 pm
- 16:00 pm
- 17:00 pm
- 18:00 pm
- 19:00 pm
- 20:00 pm
- 21:00 pm
- 22:00 pm

DAILY CHECK LIST

- ○ FOLLOW A DIET
- ○ 45 Min WORKOUT
- ○ 4 LITRES WATER
- ○ 10 PAGES READING
- ○ 5 Min COLD SHOWER
- ○ NO ALCOHOL & CHEAT MEAL
- ○ ONE ACT OF KINDNESS

TO DO LIST

○
○
○
○
○
○
○
○
○
○
○
○

DIET PLAN	BREAKFAST	
	LUNCH	
	DINNER	

WORKOUT PLAN	EXERCISE	REPETITION	DURATION	NOTES

READING	TITLE	AUTHOR	PAGES

MOOD TRACKER

WATER INTAKE

AN ACT OF KINDNESS I DID TODAY:

DATE: _____

Daily Schedule

DAY 62

DAILY SCHEDULE

- 6:00 am
- 7:00 am
- 8:00 am
- 9:00 am
- 10:00 am
- 11:00 am
- 12:00 am
- 13:00 pm
- 14:00 pm
- 15:00 pm
- 16:00 pm
- 17:00 pm
- 18:00 pm
- 19:00 pm
- 20:00 pm
- 21:00 pm
- 22:00 pm

DAILY CHECK LIST

- ○ FOLLOW A DIET
- ○ 45 Min WORKOUT
- ○ 4 LITRES WATER
- ○ 10 PAGES READING
- ○ 5 Min COLD SHOWER
- ○ NO ALCOHOL & CHEAT MEAL
- ○ ONE ACT OF KINDNESS

TO DO LIST

- ○
- ○
- ○
- ○
- ○
- ○
- ○
- ○
- ○
- ○
- ○
- ○

DIET PLAN

BREAKFAST	
LUNCH	
DINNER	

WORKOUT PLAN

EXERCISE	REPETITION	DURATION	NOTES

READING

TITLE	AUTHOR	PAGES

MOOD TRACKER

WATER INTAKE

AN ACT OF KINDNESS I DID TODAY:

DATE: .... # Daily Schedule DAY 63

DAILY SCHEDULE

6:00 am
7:00 am
8:00 am
9:00 am
10:00 am
11:00 am
12:00 am
13:00 pm
14:00 pm
15:00 pm
16:00 pm
17:00 pm
18:00 pm
19:00 pm
20:00 pm
21:00 pm
22:00 pm

DAILY CHECK LIST

- ○ FOLLOW A DIET
- ○ 45 Min WORKOUT
- ○ 4 LITRES WATER
- ○ 10 PAGES READING
- ○ 5 Min COLD SHOWER
- ○ NO ALCOHOL & CHEAT MEAL
- ○ ONE ACT OF KINDNESS

TO DO LIST

○
○
○
○
○
○
○
○
○
○
○
○

DIET PLAN

BREAKFAST	
LUNCH	
DINNER	

WORKOUT PLAN

EXERCISE	REPETITION	DURATION	NOTES

READING

TITLE	AUTHOR	PAGES

MOOD TRACKER

WATER INTAKE

AN ACT OF KINDNESS I DID TODAY:

DATE: _____ # Daily Schedule   DAY 64

DAILY SCHEDULE

- 6:00 am
- 7:00 am
- 8:00 am
- 9:00 am
- 10:00 am
- 11:00 am
- 12:00 am
- 13:00 pm
- 14:00 pm
- 15:00 pm
- 16:00 pm
- 17:00 pm
- 18:00 pm
- 19:00 pm
- 20:00 pm
- 21:00 pm
- 22:00 pm

DAILY CHECK LIST

- ○ FOLLOW A DIET
- ○ 45 Min WORKOUT
- ○ 4 LITRES WATER
- ○ 10 PAGES READING
- ○ 5 Min COLD SHOWER
- ○ NO ALCOHOL & CHEAT MEAL
- ○ ONE ACT OF KINDNESS

TO DO LIST

- ○
- ○
- ○
- ○
- ○
- ○
- ○
- ○
- ○
- ○
- ○
- ○

DIET PLAN

BREAKFAST	
LUNCH	
DINNER	

WORKOUT PLAN

EXERCISE	REPETITION	DURATION	NOTES

READING

TITLE	AUTHOR	PAGES

MOOD TRACKER

WATER INTAKE

1L 1L 1L 1L

AN ACT OF KINDNESS I DID TODAY:

DATE: ....

Daily Schedule

DAY 65

DAILY SCHEDULE

6:00 am	
7:00 am	
8:00 am	
9:00 am	
10:00 am	
11:00 am	
12:00 am	
13:00 pm	
14:00 pm	
15:00 pm	
16:00 pm	
17:00 pm	
18:00 pm	
19:00 pm	
20:00 pm	
21:00 pm	
22:00 pm	

DAILY CHECK LIST

- ○ FOLLOW A DIET
- ○ 45 Min WORKOUT
- ○ 4 LITRES WATER
- ○ 10 PAGES READING
- ○ 5 Min COLD SHOWER
- ○ NO ALCOHOL & CHEAT MEAL
- ○ ONE ACT OF KINDNESS

TO DO LIST

- ○
- ○
- ○
- ○
- ○
- ○
- ○
- ○
- ○
- ○
- ○
- ○

DIET PLAN		
	BREAKFAST	
	LUNCH	
	DINNER	

WORKOUT PLAN				
	EXERCISE	REPETITION	DURATION	NOTES

READING			
	TITLE	AUTHOR	PAGES

MOOD TRACKER

WATER INTAKE

AN ACT OF KINDNESS I DID TODAY:

Daily Schedule

DATE: _____   DAY 66

DAILY SCHEDULE

- 6:00 am
- 7:00 am
- 8:00 am
- 9:00 am
- 10:00 am
- 11:00 am
- 12:00 am
- 13:00 pm
- 14:00 pm
- 15:00 pm
- 16:00 pm
- 17:00 pm
- 18:00 pm
- 19:00 pm
- 20:00 pm
- 21:00 pm
- 22:00 pm

DAILY CHECK LIST

- ○ FOLLOW A DIET
- ○ 45 Min WORKOUT
- ○ 4 LITRES WATER
- ○ 10 PAGES READING
- ○ 5 Min COLD SHOWER
- ○ NO ALCOHOL & CHEAT MEAL
- ○ ONE ACT OF KINDNESS

TO DO LIST

- ○
- ○
- ○
- ○
- ○
- ○
- ○
- ○
- ○
- ○
- ○
- ○
- ○

DIET PLAN		
	BREAKFAST	
	LUNCH	
	DINNER	

WORKOUT PLAN				
	EXERCISE	REPETITION	DURATION	NOTES

READING			
	TITLE	AUTHOR	PAGES

MOOD TRACKER

WATER INTAKE

AN ACT OF KINDNESS I DID TODAY:

DATE: ....

Daily Schedule

DAY 67

DAILY SCHEDULE

- 6:00 am
- 7:00 am
- 8:00 am
- 9:00 am
- 10:00 am
- 11:00 am
- 12:00 am
- 13:00 pm
- 14:00 pm
- 15:00 pm
- 16:00 pm
- 17:00 pm
- 18:00 pm
- 19:00 pm
- 20:00 pm
- 21:00 pm
- 22:00 pm

DAILY CHECK LIST

- ○ FOLLOW A DIET
- ○ 45 Min WORKOUT
- ○ 4 LITRES WATER
- ○ 10 PAGES READING
- ○ 5 Min COLD SHOWER
- ○ NO ALCOHOL & CHEAT MEAL
- ○ ONE ACT OF KINDNESS

TO DO LIST

- ○
- ○
- ○
- ○
- ○
- ○
- ○
- ○
- ○
- ○
- ○
- ○

DIET PLAN

BREAKFAST	
LUNCH	
DINNER	

WORKOUT PLAN

EXERCISE	REPETITION	DURATION	NOTES

READING

TITLE	AUTHOR	PAGES

MOOD TRACKER

WATER INTAKE

AN ACT OF KINDNESS I DID TODAY:

DATE: _____ # Daily Schedule DAY 68

DAILY SCHEDULE

- 6:00 am
- 7:00 am
- 8:00 am
- 9:00 am
- 10:00 am
- 11:00 am
- 12:00 am
- 13:00 pm
- 14:00 pm
- 15:00 pm
- 16:00 pm
- 17:00 pm
- 18:00 pm
- 19:00 pm
- 20:00 pm
- 21:00 pm
- 22:00 pm

DAILY CHECK LIST

- ○ FOLLOW A DIET
- ○ 45 Min WORKOUT
- ○ 4 LITRES WATER
- ○ 10 PAGES READING
- ○ 5 Min COLD SHOWER
- ○ NO ALCOHOL & CHEAT MEAL
- ○ ONE ACT OF KINDNESS

TO DO LIST

- ○
- ○
- ○
- ○
- ○
- ○
- ○
- ○
- ○
- ○
- ○
- ○

DIET PLAN

BREAKFAST	
LUNCH	
DINNER	

WORKOUT PLAN

EXERCISE	REPETITION	DURATION	NOTES

READING

TITLE	AUTHOR	PAGES

MOOD TRACKER

WATER INTAKE

1L 1L 1L 1L

AN ACT OF KINDNESS I DID TODAY:

DATE: .... # Daily Schedule

DAILY SCHEDULE

- 6:00 am
- 7:00 am
- 8:00 am
- 9:00 am
- 10:00 am
- 11:00 am
- 12:00 am
- 13:00 pm
- 14:00 pm
- 15:00 pm
- 16:00 pm
- 17:00 pm
- 18:00 pm
- 19:00 pm
- 20:00 pm
- 21:00 pm
- 22:00 pm

DAILY CHECK LIST

- ○ FOLLOW A DIET
- ○ 45 Min WORKOUT
- ○ 4 LITRES WATER
- ○ 10 PAGES READING
- ○ 5 Min COLD SHOWER
- ○ NO ALCOHOL & CHEAT MEAL
- ○ ONE ACT OF KINDNESS

TO DO LIST

- ○
- ○
- ○
- ○
- ○
- ○
- ○
- ○
- ○
- ○
- ○

DIET PLAN

BREAKFAST		
LUNCH		
DINNER		

WORKOUT PLAN

EXERCISE	REPETITION	DURATION	NOTES

READING

TITLE	AUTHOR	PAGES

MOOD TRACKER

WATER INTAKE

AN ACT OF KINDNESS I DID TODAY:

DATE: _____ # Daily Schedule   DAY 70

DAILY SCHEDULE

- 6:00 am
- 7:00 am
- 8:00 am
- 9:00 am
- 10:00 am
- 11:00 am
- 12:00 am
- 13:00 pm
- 14:00 pm
- 15:00 pm
- 16:00 pm
- 17:00 pm
- 18:00 pm
- 19:00 pm
- 20:00 pm
- 21:00 pm
- 22:00 pm

DAILY CHECK LIST

- ○ FOLLOW A DIET
- ○ 45 Min WORKOUT
- ○ 4 LITRES WATER
- ○ 10 PAGES READING
- ○ 5 Min COLD SHOWER
- ○ NO ALCOHOL & CHEAT MEAL
- ○ ONE ACT OF KINDNESS

TO DO LIST

- ○
- ○
- ○
- ○
- ○
- ○
- ○
- ○
- ○
- ○
- ○
- ○

DIET PLAN

BREAKFAST	
LUNCH	
DINNER	

WORKOUT PLAN

EXERCISE	REPETITION	DURATION	NOTES

READING

TITLE	AUTHOR	PAGES

MOOD TRACKER

WATER INTAKE

AN ACT OF KINDNESS I DID TODAY:

DATE: _____

Daily Schedule

 DAY 71

DAILY SCHEDULE

6:00 am ....
7:00 am ....
8:00 am ....
9:00 am ....
10:00 am ....
11:00 am ....
12:00 am ....
13:00 pm ....
14:00 pm ....
15:00 pm ....
16:00 pm ....
17:00 pm ....
18:00 pm ....
19:00 pm ....
20:00 pm ....
21:00 pm ....
22:00 pm ....

DAILY CHECK LIST

- ○ FOLLOW A DIET
- ○ 45 Min WORKOUT
- ○ 4 LITRES WATER
- ○ 10 PAGES READING
- ○ 5 Min COLD SHOWER
- ○ NO ALCOHOL & CHEAT MEAL
- ○ ONE ACT OF KINDNESS

TO DO LIST

- ○ ....
- ○ ....
- ○ ....
- ○ ....
- ○ ....
- ○ ....
- ○ ....
- ○ ....
- ○ ....
- ○ ....
- ○ ....
- ○ ....

DIET PLAN

BREAKFAST	
LUNCH	
DINNER	

WORKOUT PLAN

EXERCISE	REPETITION	DURATION	NOTES

READING

TITLE	AUTHOR	PAGES

MOOD TRACKER

WATER INTAKE

AN ACT OF KINDNESS I DID TODAY:

DATE: _____

Daily Schedule

DAY 72

DAILY SCHEDULE

- 6:00 am
- 7:00 am
- 8:00 am
- 9:00 am
- 10:00 am
- 11:00 am
- 12:00 am
- 13:00 pm
- 14:00 pm
- 15:00 pm
- 16:00 pm
- 17:00 pm
- 18:00 pm
- 19:00 pm
- 20:00 pm
- 21:00 pm
- 22:00 pm

DAILY CHECK LIST

- ○ FOLLOW A DIET
- ○ 45 Min WORKOUT
- ○ 4 LITRES WATER
- ○ 10 PAGES READING
- ○ 5 Min COLD SHOWER
- ○ NO ALCOHOL & CHEAT MEAL
- ○ ONE ACT OF KINDNESS

TO DO LIST

- ○
- ○
- ○
- ○
- ○
- ○
- ○
- ○
- ○
- ○
- ○
- ○

DIET PLAN

BREAKFAST	
LUNCH	
DINNER	

WORKOUT PLAN

EXERCISE	REPETITION	DURATION	NOTES

READING

TITLE	AUTHOR	PAGES

MOOD TRACKER

WATER INTAKE

1L 1L 1L 1L

AN ACT OF KINDNESS I DID TODAY:

Daily Schedule

DATE: ....

DAY 73

DAILY SCHEDULE

- 6:00 am
- 7:00 am
- 8:00 am
- 9:00 am
- 10:00 am
- 11:00 am
- 12:00 am
- 13:00 pm
- 14:00 pm
- 15:00 pm
- 16:00 pm
- 17:00 pm
- 18:00 pm
- 19:00 pm
- 20:00 pm
- 21:00 pm
- 22:00 pm

DAILY CHECK LIST

- ○ FOLLOW A DIET
- ○ 45 Min WORKOUT
- ○ 4 LITRES WATER
- ○ 10 PAGES READING
- ○ 5 Min COLD SHOWER
- ○ NO ALCOHOL & CHEAT MEAL
- ○ ONE ACT OF KINDNESS

TO DO LIST

- ○
- ○
- ○
- ○
- ○
- ○
- ○
- ○
- ○
- ○
- ○
- ○

DIET PLAN

BREAKFAST	
LUNCH	
DINNER	

WORKOUT PLAN

EXERCISE	REPETITION	DURATION	NOTES

READING

TITLE	AUTHOR	PAGES

MOOD TRACKER

WATER INTAKE

AN ACT OF KINDNESS I DID TODAY:

DATE: _____ # Daily Schedule

DAILY SCHEDULE

- 6:00 am
- 7:00 am
- 8:00 am
- 9:00 am
- 10:00 am
- 11:00 am
- 12:00 am
- 13:00 pm
- 14:00 pm
- 15:00 pm
- 16:00 pm
- 17:00 pm
- 18:00 pm
- 19:00 pm
- 20:00 pm
- 21:00 pm
- 22:00 pm

DAILY CHECK LIST

- ○ FOLLOW A DIET
- ○ 45 Min WORKOUT
- ○ 4 LITRES WATER
- ○ 10 PAGES READING
- ○ 5 Min COLD SHOWER
- ○ NO ALCOHOL & CHEAT MEAL
- ○ ONE ACT OF KINDNESS

TO DO LIST

- ○
- ○
- ○
- ○
- ○
- ○
- ○
- ○
- ○
- ○
- ○

DIET PLAN

BREAKFAST	
LUNCH	
DINNER	

WORKOUT PLAN

EXERCISE	REPETITION	DURATION	NOTES

READING

TITLE	AUTHOR	PAGES

MOOD TRACKER

WATER INTAKE

AN ACT OF KINDNESS I DID TODAY:

DATE: .... # Daily Schedule   DAY 75

DAILY SCHEDULE

- 6:00 am
- 7:00 am
- 8:00 am
- 9:00 am
- 10:00 am
- 11:00 am
- 12:00 am
- 13:00 pm
- 14:00 pm
- 15:00 pm
- 16:00 pm
- 17:00 pm
- 18:00 pm
- 19:00 pm
- 20:00 pm
- 21:00 pm
- 22:00 pm

DAILY CHECK LIST

- ○ FOLLOW A DIET
- ○ 45 Min WORKOUT
- ○ 4 LITRES WATER
- ○ 10 PAGES READING
- ○ 5 Min COLD SHOWER
- ○ NO ALCOHOL & CHEAT MEAL
- ○ ONE ACT OF KINDNESS

TO DO LIST

- ○
- ○
- ○
- ○
- ○
- ○
- ○
- ○
- ○
- ○
- ○
- ○
- ○

DIET PLAN

BREAKFAST	
LUNCH	
DINNER	

WORKOUT PLAN

EXERCISE	REPETITION	DURATION	NOTES

READING

TITLE	AUTHOR	PAGES

MOOD TRACKER

WATER INTAKE

AN ACT OF KINDNESS I DID TODAY:

Copyrights 2022 - All rights reserved

You may not reproduce, duplicate, or send the contents of this book without direct written permission from the author. You cannot hereby despite any circumstance blame the publisher or hold him or her the legal responsibility for any reparation, compensation or monetary forfeiture owing to the information included herein, either in a direct or indirect way.

Legal Notice: This book has copyright protection. You can use the book for personal purpose. You should not sell, use, alter, distribute, quote, take excerpts or paraphrase in part of whole the material contained in this book without obtaining the permission of the author first.

Disclaimer Notice: You must take note that the information in this document is for casual reading and entertainment purpose only. We have made every attempt to provide accurate, up to date and reliable information. We do not express or imply guarantees of any kind. The person who read admit that the writer is not occupied in giving legal, financial, medical, or other advice. We put this book content by sourcing various places.

Please consult a licensed professional before you try any techniques shown in this book.By going through this document, the book lover comes to an agreement that under no situation is the author accountable for any forfeiture, direct or indirect, which they may incur because of the use of material contained in this document, including, but not limited to, - errors, omissions, or inaccuracies.

Thank You!

Thank you so much for trying our 75 Hard Challenge Book. We'd love to hear from you!

If you've found this to be a good book please, support us and leave a review.

If you have any suggestions or issues with this book, or if you want to test some of our latest notebooks please email us.

Send email to:

pickme.readme@gmail.com